FUCK THIS SHIT!

A Journal of Serenity, Gratitude and Sobriety.

(How to Become Happy, Joyous and Free in a World of Shit)

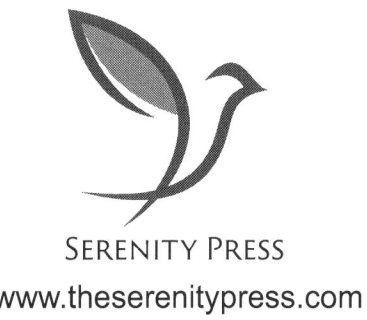

SERENITY PRESS
www.theserenitypress.com

© 2019 The Serenity Press - All Rights Reserved

When the Shit Gets Too Much To Take:
(Your Sponsor's Contact Information)

(The Time to Call is BEFORE The Shit Gets Too Much!)

When the Shit Gets Serious:
(Emergency Information)

(If You're Reading This... Help! Save My Ass!)

Where I Can Put My Shit on the Table:
(Meeting Times, Locations)

(Keep Coming Back, No Matter How Much Shit You Bring!)

This is the Kind of Shit I Have to Deal With:
(Today's Personal Inventory)

(Own Your Own Shit, Accept the Shit You Can't Change)

Did I Do That Shit?
(Your Daily Amends)

(Kindness is ALWAYS the Best Policy)

Shit That Made Me Happy:
(Today's Gratitude List)

(The Shit is not ALL Bad!)

Seriously, What The Fuck?
(Things to Discuss With Your Sponsor)

(Seriously, They Can Help You With Your Shit)

Leave That Shit Alone:
(Things I Need to Let My HP Deal With)

(Some Shit is Out of Your Hands)

Fuck 'Em:
(Things You Probably Should Not Say Out Loud)

(Restraint of Pen and Tongue ...but Go On, Get That Shit Out!)

Holy Fucking Shit:
(Today's Spiritual Growth)

(How Is That Shit Working for You Today?)

That Shit Hurts!
(This Too Shall Pass)

(You WILL Get Through This Shit)

It's a Shit Storm!
(Find Your Serenity)

(Even If the World is Going to Shit, Find Your Calm Inner Peace)

That's Some Complicated Shit!
(Keep It Simple)

(Life Can Be Pretty Fucking Confusing, Sobriety Shouldn't Be)

The Shit Hit The Fan:
(What Gives You Hope Today?)

(What Gives You Strength in a World of Shit?)

This Shit Just Got Real:
(How Did You Get Out of Self and Help Others Today?)

(Your Experience, Strength and Hope Can Help Others with Their Shit)

That's Some Good Shit:
(What Did You Do Well Today?)

(Celebrate the Good Shit You Do)

Shit Happens:
(Things I Don't Need To Worry About)

(With or Without Me, That Shit Is Going to Happen)

That's Some Scary Ass Shit:
(FEAR = Face Everything and Recover)

(It Is Just Future - Shitty - Events that APPEAR Real)

That's a Shitty Thing:
(Draw What You are Feeling)

(Your Shit Just Became Real)

Shit On The Paper:
(What's Going On In Your Head and Heart?)

(Putting That Shit on Paper Helps Work It Out)

This is the Kind of Shit I Have to Deal With:
(Today's Personal Inventory)

(Own Your Own Shit, Accept the Shit You Can't Change)

Did I Do That Shit?
(Your Daily Amends)

(Kindness is ALWAYS the Best Policy)

Shit That Made Me Happy:
(Today's Gratitude List)

(The Shit is not ALL Bad!)

Seriously, What The Fuck?
(Things to Discuss With Your Sponsor)

(Seriously, They Can Help You With Your Shit)

Leave That Shit Alone:
(Things I Need to Let My HP Deal With)

(Some Shit is Out of Your Hands)

Fuck 'Em:
(Things You Probably Should Not Say Out Loud)

(Restraint of Pen and Tongue ...but Go On, Get That Shit Out!)

Holy Fucking Shit:
(Today's Spiritual Growth)

(How Is That Shit Working for You Today?)

That Shit Hurts!
(This Too Shall Pass)

(You WILL Get Through This Shit)

It's a Shit Storm!
(Find Your Serenity)

(Even If the World is Going to Shit, Find Your Calm Inner Peace)

That's Some Complicated Shit!
(Keep It Simple)

(Life Can Be Pretty Fucking Confusing, Sobriety Shouldn't Be)

The Shit Hit The Fan:
(What Gives You Hope Today?)

(What Gives You Strength in a World of Shit?)

This Shit Just Got Real:
(How Did You Get Out of Self and Help Others Today?)

(Your Experience, Strength and Hope Can Help Others with Their Shit)

That's Some Good Shit:
(What Did You Do Well Today?)

(Celebrate the Good Shit You Do)

Shit Happens:
(Things I Don't Need To Worry About)

(With or Without Me, That Shit Is Going to Happen)

That's Some Scary Ass Shit:
(FEAR = Face Everything and Recover)

(It Is Just Future - Shitty - Events that APPEAR Real)

That's a Shitty Thing:
(Draw What You are Feeling)

(Your Shit Just Became Real)

Shit On The Paper:
(What's Going On In Your Head and Heart?)

(Putting That Shit on Paper Helps Work It Out)

This is the Kind of Shit I Have to Deal With:
(Today's Personal Inventory)

(Own Your Own Shit, Accept the Shit You Can't Change)

Did I Do That Shit?
(Your Daily Amends)

(Kindness is ALWAYS the Best Policy)

Shit That Made Me Happy:
(Today's Gratitude List)

(The Shit is not ALL Bad!)

Seriously, What The Fuck?
(Things to Discuss With Your Sponsor)

(Seriously, They Can Help You With Your Shit)

Leave That Shit Alone:
(Things I Need to Let My HP Deal With)

(Some Shit is Out of Your Hands)

Fuck 'Em:
(Things You Probably Should Not Say Out Loud)

(Restraint of Pen and Tongue ...but Go On, Get That Shit Out!)

Holy Fucking Shit:
(Today's Spiritual Growth)

(How Is That Shit Working for You Today?)

That Shit Hurts!
(This Too Shall Pass)

(You WILL Get Through This Shit)

It's a Shit Storm!
(Find Your Serenity)

(Even If the World is Going to Shit, Find Your Calm Inner Peace)

That's Some Complicated Shit!
(Keep It Simple)

(Life Can Be Pretty Fucking Confusing, Sobriety Shouldn't Be)

The Shit Hit The Fan:
(What Gives You Hope Today?)

(What Gives You Strength in a World of Shit?)

This Shit Just Got Real:
(How Did You Get Out of Self and Help Others Today?)

(Your Experience, Strength and Hope Can Help Others with Their Shit)

That's Some Good Shit:
(What Did You Do Well Today?)

(Celebrate the Good Shit You Do)

Shit Happens:
(Things I Don't Need To Worry About)

(With or Without Me, That Shit Is Going to Happen)

That's Some Scary Ass Shit:
(FEAR = Face Everything and Recover)

(It Is Just Future - Shitty - Events that APPEAR Real)

That's a Shitty Thing:
(Draw What You are Feeling)

(Your Shit Just Became Real)

Shit On The Paper:
(What's Going On In Your Head and Heart?)

(Putting That Shit on Paper Helps Work It Out)

Did I Do That Shit?
(Your Daily Amends)

(Kindness is ALWAYS the Best Policy)

Shit That Made Me Happy:
(Today's Gratitude List)

(The Shit is not ALL Bad!)

Seriously, What The Fuck?
(Things to Discuss With Your Sponsor)

(Seriously, They Can Help You With Your Shit)

Leave That Shit Alone:
(Things I Need to Let My HP Deal With)

(Some Shit is Out of Your Hands)

Fuck 'Em:
(Things You Probably Should Not Say Out Loud)

(Restraint of Pen and Tongue ...but Go On, Get That Shit Out!)

Holy Fucking Shit:
(Today's Spiritual Growth)

(How Is That Shit Working for You Today?)

That Shit Hurts!
(This Too Shall Pass)

(You WILL Get Through This Shit)

It's a Shit Storm!
(Find Your Serenity)

(Even If the World is Going to Shit, Find Your Calm Inner Peace)

That's Some Complicated Shit!
(Keep It Simple)

(Life Can Be Pretty Fucking Confusing, Sobriety Shouldn't Be)

The Shit Hit The Fan:
(What Gives You Hope Today?)

(What Gives You Strength in a World of Shit?)

This Shit Just Got Real:
(How Did You Get Out of Self and Help Others Today?)

(Your Experience, Strength and Hope Can Help Others with Their Shit)

That's Some Good Shit:
(What Did You Do Well Today?)

(Celebrate the Good Shit You Do)

Shit Happens:
(Things I Don't Need To Worry About)

(With or Without Me, That Shit Is Going to Happen)

That's Some Scary Ass Shit:
(FEAR = Face Everything and Recover)

(It Is Just Future - Shitty - Events that APPEAR Real)

That's a Shitty Thing:
(Draw What You are Feeling)

(Your Shit Just Became Real)

Shit On The Paper:
(What's Going On In Your Head and Heart?)

(Putting That Shit on Paper Helps Work It Out)

Did I Do That Shit?
(Your Daily Amends)

(Kindness is ALWAYS the Best Policy)

Shit That Made Me Happy:
(Today's Gratitude List)

(The Shit is not ALL Bad!)

Seriously, What The Fuck?
(Things to Discuss With Your Sponsor)

(Seriously, They Can Help You With Your Shit)

Leave That Shit Alone:
(Things I Need to Let My HP Deal With)

(Some Shit is Out of Your Hands)

Fuck 'Em:
(Things You Probably Should Not Say Out Loud)

(Restraint of Pen and Tongue ...but Go On, Get That Shit Out!)

Holy Fucking Shit:
(Today's Spiritual Growth)

(How Is That Shit Working for You Today?)

That Shit Hurts!
(This Too Shall Pass)

(You WILL Get Through This Shit)

It's a Shit Storm!
(Find Your Serenity)

(Even If the World is Going to Shit, Find Your Calm Inner Peace)

That's Some Complicated Shit!
(Keep It Simple)

(Life Can Be Pretty Fucking Confusing, Sobriety Shouldn't Be)

The Shit Hit The Fan:
(What Gives You Hope Today?)

(What Gives You Strength in a World of Shit?)

This Shit Just Got Real:
(How Did You Get Out of Self and Help Others Today?)

(Your Experience, Strength and Hope Can Help Others with Their Shit)

That's Some Good Shit:
(What Did You Do Well Today?)

(Celebrate the Good Shit You Do)

Shit Happens:
(Things I Don't Need To Worry About)

(With or Without Me, That Shit Is Going to Happen)

That's Some Scary Ass Shit:
(FEAR = Face Everything and Recover)

(It Is Just Future - Shitty - Events that APPEAR Real)

That's a Shitty Thing:
(Draw What You are Feeling)

(Your Shit Just Became Real)

Shit On The Paper:
(What's Going On In Your Head and Heart?)

(Putting That Shit on Paper Helps Work It Out)

This is the Kind of Shit I Have to Deal With:
(Today's Personal Inventory)

(Own Your Own Shit, Accept the Shit You Can't Change)

Did I Do That Shit?
(Your Daily Amends)

(Kindness is ALWAYS the Best Policy)

Shit That Made Me Happy:
(Today's Gratitude List)

(The Shit is not ALL Bad!)

Seriously, What The Fuck?
(Things to Discuss With Your Sponsor)

(Seriously, They Can Help You With Your Shit)

Leave That Shit Alone:
(Things I Need to Let My HP Deal With)

(Some Shit is Out of Your Hands)

Fuck 'Em:
(Things You Probably Should Not Say Out Loud)

(Restraint of Pen and Tongue ...but Go On, Get That Shit Out!)

Holy Fucking Shit:
(Today's Spiritual Growth)

(How Is That Shit Working for You Today?)

That Shit Hurts!
(This Too Shall Pass)

(You WILL Get Through This Shit)

It's a Shit Storm!
(Find Your Serenity)

(Even If the World is Going to Shit, Find Your Calm Inner Peace)

That's Some Complicated Shit!
(Keep It Simple)

(Life Can Be Pretty Fucking Confusing, Sobriety Shouldn't Be)

The Shit Hit The Fan:
(What Gives You Hope Today?)

(What Gives You Strength in a World of Shit?)

This Shit Just Got Real:
(How Did You Get Out of Self and Help Others Today?)

(Your Experience, Strength and Hope Can Help Others with Their Shit)

That's Some Good Shit:
(What Did You Do Well Today?)

(Celebrate the Good Shit You Do)

Shit Happens:
(Things I Don't Need To Worry About)

(With or Without Me, That Shit Is Going to Happen)

That's Some Scary Ass Shit:
(FEAR = Face Everything and Recover)

(It Is Just Future - Shitty - Events that APPEAR Real)

That's a Shitty Thing:
(Draw What You are Feeling)

(Your Shit Just Became Real)

Shit On The Paper:
(What's Going On In Your Head and Heart?)

(Putting That Shit on Paper Helps Work It Out)

This is the Kind of Shit I Have to Deal With:
(Today's Personal Inventory)

(Own Your Own Shit, Accept the Shit You Can't Change)

Did I Do That Shit?
(Your Daily Amends)

(Kindness is ALWAYS the Best Policy)

Shit That Made Me Happy:
(Today's Gratitude List)

(The Shit is not ALL Bad!)

Seriously, What The Fuck?
(Things to Discuss With Your Sponsor)

(Seriously, They Can Help You With Your Shit)

Leave That Shit Alone:
(Things I Need to Let My HP Deal With)

(Some Shit is Out of Your Hands)

Fuck 'Em:
(Things You Probably Should Not Say Out Loud)

(Restraint of Pen and Tongue ...but Go On, Get That Shit Out!)

Holy Fucking Shit:
(Today's Spiritual Growth)

(How Is That Shit Working for You Today?)

That Shit Hurts!
(This Too Shall Pass)

(You WILL Get Through This Shit)

It's a Shit Storm!
(Find Your Serenity)

(Even If the World is Going to Shit, Find Your Calm Inner Peace)

That's Some Complicated Shit!
(Keep It Simple)

(Life Can Be Pretty Fucking Confusing, Sobriety Shouldn't Be)

The Shit Hit The Fan:
(What Gives You Hope Today?)

(What Gives You Strength in a World of Shit?)

This Shit Just Got Real:
(How Did You Get Out of Self and Help Others Today?)

(Your Experience, Strength and Hope Can Help Others with Their Shit)

That's Some Good Shit:
(What Did You Do Well Today?)

(Celebrate the Good Shit You Do)

Shit Happens:
(Things I Don't Need To Worry About)

(With or Without Me, That Shit Is Going to Happen)

That's Some Scary Ass Shit:
(FEAR = Face Everything and Recover)

(It Is Just Future - Shitty - Events that APPEAR Real)

That's a Shitty Thing:
(Draw What You are Feeling)

(Your Shit Just Became Real)

Shit On The Paper:
(What's Going On In Your Head and Heart?)

(Putting That Shit on Paper Helps Work It Out)

This is the Kind of Shit I Have to Deal With:
(Today's Personal Inventory)

(Own Your Own Shit, Accept the Shit You Can't Change)

Did I Do That Shit?
(Your Daily Amends)

(Kindness is ALWAYS the Best Policy)

Shit That Made Me Happy:
(Today's Gratitude List)

(The Shit is not ALL Bad!)

Seriously, What The Fuck?
(Things to Discuss With Your Sponsor)

(Seriously, They Can Help You With Your Shit)

Leave That Shit Alone:
(Things I Need to Let My HP Deal With)

(Some Shit is Out of Your Hands)

Fuck 'Em:
(Things You Probably Should Not Say Out Loud)

(Restraint of Pen and Tongue ...but Go On, Get That Shit Out!)

Holy Fucking Shit:
(Today's Spiritual Growth)

(How Is That Shit Working for You Today?)

That Shit Hurts!
(This Too Shall Pass)

(You WILL Get Through This Shit)

It's a Shit Storm!
(Find Your Serenity)

(Even If the World is Going to Shit, Find Your Calm Inner Peace)

That's Some Complicated Shit!
(Keep It Simple)

(Life Can Be Pretty Fucking Confusing, Sobriety Shouldn't Be)

The Shit Hit The Fan:
(What Gives You Hope Today?)

(What Gives You Strength in a World of Shit?)

This Shit Just Got Real:
(How Did You Get Out of Self and Help Others Today?)

(Your Experience, Strength and Hope Can Help Others with Their Shit)

That's Some Good Shit:
(What Did You Do Well Today?)

(Celebrate the Good Shit You Do)

Shit Happens:
(Things I Don't Need To Worry About)

(With or Without Me, That Shit Is Going to Happen)

That's Some Scary Ass Shit:
(FEAR = Face Everything and Recover)

(It Is Just Future - Shitty - Events that APPEAR Real)

That's a Shitty Thing:
(Draw What You are Feeling)

(Your Shit Just Became Real)

Shit On The Paper:
(What's Going On In Your Head and Heart?)

(Putting That Shit on Paper Helps Work It Out)

This is the Kind of Shit I Have to Deal With:
(Today's Personal Inventory)

(Own Your Own Shit, Accept the Shit You Can't Change)

Did I Do That Shit?
(Your Daily Amends)

(Kindness is ALWAYS the Best Policy)

Shit That Made Me Happy:
(Today's Gratitude List)

(The Shit is not ALL Bad!)

Seriously, What The Fuck?
(Things to Discuss With Your Sponsor)

(Seriously, They Can Help You With Your Shit)

Leave That Shit Alone:
(Things I Need to Let My HP Deal With)

(Some Shit is Out of Your Hands)

Fuck 'Em:
(Things You Probably Should Not Say Out Loud)

(Restraint of Pen and Tongue ...but Go On, Get That Shit Out!)

Holy Fucking Shit:
(Today's Spiritual Growth)

(How Is That Shit Working for You Today?)

That Shit Hurts!
(This Too Shall Pass)

(You WILL Get Through This Shit)

It's a Shit Storm!
(Find Your Serenity)

(Even If the World is Going to Shit, Find Your Calm Inner Peace)

That's Some Complicated Shit!
(Keep It Simple)

(Life Can Be Pretty Fucking Confusing, Sobriety Shouldn't Be)

The Shit Hit The Fan:
(What Gives You Hope Today?)

(What Gives You Strength in a World of Shit?)

This Shit Just Got Real:
(How Did You Get Out of Self and Help Others Today?)

(Your Experience, Strength and Hope Can Help Others with Their Shit)

That's Some Good Shit:
(What Did You Do Well Today?)

(Celebrate the Good Shit You Do)

Shit Happens:
(Things I Don't Need To Worry About)

(With or Without Me, That Shit Is Going to Happen)

That's Some Scary Ass Shit:
(FEAR = Face Everything and Recover)

(It Is Just Future - Shitty - Events that APPEAR Real)

That's a Shitty Thing:
(Draw What You are Feeling)

(Your Shit Just Became Real)

Shit On The Paper:
(What's Going On In Your Head and Heart?)

(Putting That Shit on Paper Helps Work It Out)

Made in the USA
Lexington, KY
27 February 2019